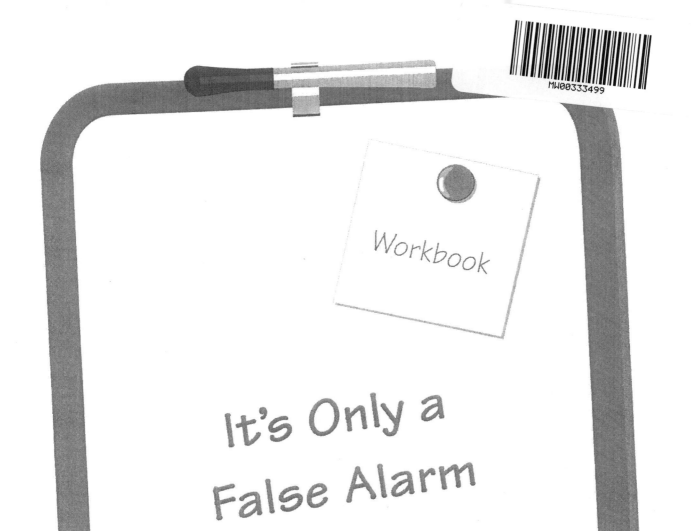

Workbook

It's Only a False Alarm

John Piacentini · Audra Langley · Tami Roblek

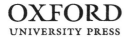

UNIVERSITY PRESS

2007

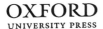

Oxford University Press, Inc., publishes works that further
Oxford University's objective of excellence
in research, scholarship, and education.

Oxford   New York
Auckland   Cape Town   Dar es Salaam   Hong Kong   Karachi
Kuala Lumpur   Madrid   Melbourne   Mexico City   Nairobi
New Delhi   Shanghai   Taipei   Toronto

With offices in
Argentina   Austria   Brazil   Chile   Czech Republic   France   Greece
Guatemala   Hungary   Italy   Japan   Poland   Portugal   Singapore
South Korea   Switzerland   Thailand   Turkey   Ukraine   Vietnam

Copyright © 2007 by Oxford University Press, Inc.

Published by Oxford University Press, Inc.
198 Madison Avenue, New York, New York 10016

www.oup.com

Oxford is a registered trademark of Oxford University Press

ISBN 978-0-19-531052-8

9 8 7 6 5 4 3 2

Printed in the United States of America

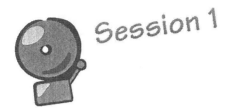 *Session 1*

 *Chapter 1*

Welcome!

Welcome to the "It's Only a False Alarm" program! You and your therapist will use this workbook together to learn how to deal with the problems you are having with your thoughts and behaviors—a problem known as *obsessive–compulsive disorder* or *OCD*. You will use this workbook each time you visit your therapist. Each visit is called a *session*. During this first session, your therapist will talk to you and your family about OCD and how this program works to help children feel better. During the next session, your therapist will work with you and your family to better understand how OCD affects your life and to create a specific plan to help you fight this problem.

Your plan will include learning new skills to help you face the things that make you nervous or scared. This is called *exposure practice* and you will do this in every session. You and your therapist will work as a team to decide which things to practice each week, starting with your least scary thoughts and behaviors first. The more you use the plan, the better your OCD will get. By the end of the program, your OCD should be much better or even completely gone! This workbook is divided into 12 sessions. Some kids need more than 12 sessions; others need less. You and your therapist will decide the right number of sessions for you and the best way to use this workbook.

Your family will be with you throughout this program. Your therapist will meet with them, as well, and will teach them the best ways to help you get better.

The first thing your therapist will do is explain to you what OCD is.

What Is Obsessive–Compulsive Disorder?

Obsessive–compulsive disorder is also known as OCD. If you have OCD, you probably worry a lot and feel nervous and scared sometimes. Maybe you are afraid to touch certain things because you think they are dirty or covered with germs. Maybe you worry that something bad will happen to you or to someone you love. These kinds of negative thoughts are called *obsessions* and they make up the "O" part of OCD.

Obsessions are the thoughts, images, urges, feelings, or sensations that you have that make you feel anxious or upset or "icky." Like we just talked about, these thoughts can be about things being dirty or covered with germs, about bad things happening to you or other people, or just a feeling that something is wrong or not quite right. People with these thoughts usually don't want to have them and try to make them go away by doing certain things, like washing their hands a lot, counting, repeating, checking things over and over, or other special things that make them feel better. Sometimes these thoughts or feelings make kids want to do something over and over again until they feel "just right" or "complete."

Do you have thoughts that make you feel nervous or worried? Some kids call these thoughts their "worries," "icky thoughts," "OCD thoughts," or "scary thoughts."

What do you call your OCD thoughts?

_____

Write some of them down in the blanks provided.

My Obsessions:

1. _____

2. _____

3. _____

4. _____

5. _____

Do you do special things to make your bad thoughts go away? The things you do, like counting and checking over and over again, are called *compulsions* and they make up the "C" part of OCD. Compulsions are things like washing your hands or other things over and over, checking or repeating things, or saying things in a certain way or a certain number of times. Sometimes kids call their compulsions by different names, like "habits," "phobias," "rituals," or "tricks."

My Compulsions:

1. _____

2. _____

3. _____

4. _____

5. _____

OCD Is Like a False Fire Alarm

We can use the example of a fire alarm to understand how OCD works. Have you ever heard the fire alarm go off at your school or in another public place? The loud ringing sound and teachers telling you to leave the school can make you anxious so you will want to leave the building and go to a safe place. However, sometimes the fire alarm goes off when there is no fire, either by accident or maybe someone is playing a trick. Even though there is no fire, the bells ring and people get a little anxious and leave the building to be safe. People think there is something dangerous happening, but there really isn't. OCD is like a false fire alarm. When someone with OCD gets an obsession or scary thought, it's like someone pulled a fire alarm in your head. It makes the person feel nervous or that something bad is going to happen. However, just like a false fire alarm, there is nothing really dangerous around. We will use a kind of treatment called *cognitive-behavior therapy,* or CBT, to treat your OCD. In CBT, you will learn how to tell that your OCD fears are false alarms and that nothing bad will happen if you ignore them.

Other Kids Have OCD, Too

Did you know that, on average, one or two kids out of every hundred has OCD? That's a lot of people. Do you know anybody in your school or from somewhere else who has OCD or who you think may have OCD? You may not know very many of these other kids with OCD because most of them are probably trying to keep it secret just like you. We can figure out about how many kids in your school might have OCD; I'll bet you will be surprised by the number.

How Many Kids Have OCD?

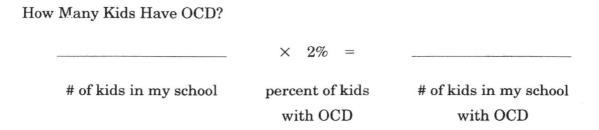

| _____ | × 2% = | _____ |
| # of kids in my school | percent of kids with OCD | # of kids in my school with OCD |

I'll bet you also didn't know that everybody has strange, scary, or weird thoughts sometimes. The problem is that, even though these thoughts aren't real, OCD can make them get stuck in your head and still make you feel really worried or bad about them.

What Causes OCD?

For most people, OCD is thought to be a medical condition. Our bodies are made up of a lot of different chemicals that control all of the things we do, like eating, sleeping, running fast, thinking, and feeling. Each person has slightly different amounts of these chemicals in their bodies. That's one of the things that makes each one of us different from everyone else. Some doctors and scientists think that people with OCD may have just a little bit more or less of some of these chemicals, including a chemical called *serotonin,* than other people. This may be one of the reasons people with OCD are bothered by their "false alarm" thoughts and feelings or have to do certain things more than other people. The good news is that the plan you and your therapist develop can fix this problem and help your OCD get better or go away completely.

Although some people with OCD think their problems are crazy or weird, or that they are really different from other people, having OCD is really just like having any other physical illness or problem, like asthma, diabetes, or needing to wear glasses to see, or needing braces on your teeth. People wear glasses or braces because they have a problem with their eyes or their teeth. People with asthma have a problem with how they breathe, and having diabetes means you have a problem with how your body handles sugar. In just the same way, OCD is a problem with how you control your thoughts, feelings, and behaviors. OCD is a lot like these other problems in other ways, as well. Like asthma, OCD tends to get worse when you are tired, stressed out, or physically ill. Also, OCD usually does not go away by itself, although it may get better or worse at different times. Sometimes OCD symptoms may also be related to things that have actually happened to you or other people you know. For example, getting stuck in an elevator has led some people to get really scared of elevators. In some cases, whenever they need to go on an elevator or even see an elevator, they need to do rituals like praying or counting or other things to make the bad feeling go away.

The Obsessive-Compulsive Cycle

Did you know that the more you do your rituals, the stronger they become? That's because you are actually teaching yourself to do rituals whenever you feel anxious or have false alarm thoughts and feelings. So doing rituals actually tricks you into thinking that this is the only way to make the scary or false alarm thoughts and feelings go away. The picture here (Figure 1.1) shows how doing rituals can make your OCD worse.

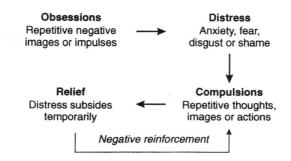

This Program

This program will help you learn to control your OCD and not feel bad when you get OCD thoughts or have to do rituals. Remember that your OCD is like a false fire alarm that makes you feel worried even when there is no fire. What do you think would happen if you had a negative thought and didn't do your ritual? Have you ever been in a situation where you wanted to do your ritual but couldn't? What happened? Write about your experience in the lines provided.

OCD might make you think that your anxiety would go higher and higher and not stop. But that's not really true. Like most people, your anxiety would probably go away by itself—although it might take a little bit longer than if you did your ritual. The more you resist giving in to your OCD "false alarm," the weaker it will get. If you practice enough, your OCD thoughts may even go away completely.

Your therapist will help you practice doing things that make you feel a little uncomfortable or anxious at first without doing your rituals. This is called *exposure and response prevention.* It's like when you first dip your toes into a swimming pool and it feels *sooo* cold! After a few minutes, though, your body gets used to the water and your toes actually start to feel comfortable. This program works the same way. Exposure practice will start with the OCD thoughts or behaviors that bother you the least. After you have practiced the easier things for a while, you will slowly move up to things that are more difficult. You and your therapist will decide together how and when to work your way up to more difficult exposures.

The Behavioral Reward Program

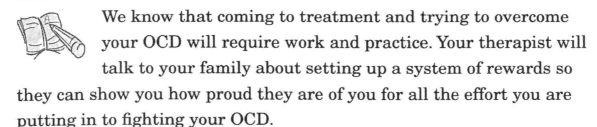 We know that coming to treatment and trying to overcome your OCD will require work and practice. Your therapist will talk to your family about setting up a system of rewards so they can show you how proud they are of you for all the effort you are putting in to fighting your OCD.

Work with your therapist and your family to brainstorm some rewards using the form provided.

My Rewards Program

What I Do:	My Reward:
_____	_____
_____	_____
_____	_____
_____	_____
_____	_____
_____	_____

Keeping Track of Your Symptoms

During your first session, your therapist will teach you how to keep track of your obsessions and compulsions using a form called *My Symptom Diary*. We have included a blank diary here, as well as an example of a completed diary (Figure 1.2) so you can use it as a model when filling out your own.

My Symptom Diary

This diary is to help you keep track of some of the OCD symptoms that you have talked about in treatment. Please write down each time that you feel like doing the symptom, each time you actually do the symptom. If your symptom happens too often to rate every time you do it, then your therapist and you will work out a specific time of day for you to keep track of it.

Symptom: _____

Date	Time	Obsession (or worry)	Compulsion

This diary is to help you keep track of some of the OCD symptoms that you have talked about during treatment. Please write down each time that you feel like doing the symptom, each time you actually do the symptom. If your symptom happens too often to rate every time you do it, then your therapist and you will work out a specific time of day for you to keep track of it.

Symptom: _Afraid to touch the bathroom doorknob_

Date	Time	Obsession (or Worry)	Compulsion
10/4	9:00 AM	Germs, getting sick	Used sleeve to open door
10/5	9:30 AM	Germs, getting sick	Washed hands after
10/5	12:20 AM	Germs, getting sick	Washed hands after
10/6	11:15 AM	Germs, getting sick	Washed hands after
10/7	8:20 AM	Germs, getting sick	Used other bathroom
10/7	3:45 PM	Germs, getting sick	Used other bathroom
10/7	9:15 PM	Germs, getting sick	Used sleeve to open door
10/8	9:25 AM	Germs, getting sick	Washed hands after
10/8	5:15 PM	Germs, getting sick	Washed hands after

Figure 1.2 **Example of Completed My Symptom Diary**

Exercises

▨ At the end of this session, your therapist may ask you to fill out a form called the CY-BOCS that will help him or her understand your symptoms. Your family may help you complete this checklist if necessary.

▨ Use the My Symptom Diary to monitor your obsessions and compulsions during the next week.

▨ Work with your family to create a program for rewarding you for your effort while participating in this program.

 Session 2

Chapter

2

OCD Thermometer

The OCD thermometer (Figure 2.1) is just like a regular thermometer only it measures anxiety and other bad feelings instead of the temperature. The high numbers represent really bad or anxious feelings (10 is the worst you've ever felt), whereas the low numbers mean that you hardly have any bad or anxious feelings at all. Zero means no anxiety at all. Can you think of some examples of things that make you have a low temperature? A medium temperature? And a high temperature? You will use the OCD thermometer to rate your OCD symptoms from the least upsetting to the most upsetting.

My Symptom List

Use the form on page 14 to list your OCD symptoms. This list will help you and your therapist to decide which symptoms to work on during each session. Remember the exposures we talked about during session 1? The symptoms on this list will be used for your exposure exercises. Remember to use your OCD thermometer to rate each of the symptoms on your list. You will start by facing the things that only bother you a little bit and work your way up, little by little, to the harder things. It's like going into the pool. First you put your feet in and get used to the water, then you go in up to your knees and, after that's comfortable, you go in a bit farther.

Hardest to resist (most scary or upsetting)

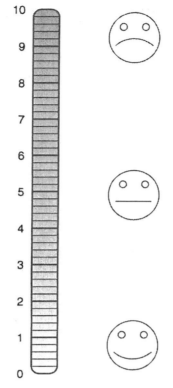

Easiest to resist (least scary or upsetting)

Figure 2.1 OCD Thermometer

You and your therapist will decide together the order of symptoms to work on. You will not have to do any exposures that you feel are too hard for you. In other words, you don't have to go into the pool up to your waist right away. You may want to wait until you are comfortable with your feet and legs in the water. At that point, going in up to your waist probably won't seem so difficult or scary anymore.

You and your therapist will talk about which exposure to start working on first. Next session, you will practice doing this exposure with your therapist.

Exercises

▓ Use the My Symptom Diary to monitor your obsessions and compulsions during the next week.

My Symptom List

Name: _____

OCD Thermometer Rating

DATE:					
SESSION:	1				
SYMPTOM:					

My Symptom Diary

This diary is to help you keep track of some of the OCD symptoms that you have talked about in treatment. Please write down each time that you feel like doing the symptom, each time you actually do the symptom, and what your OCD thermometer rating for the symptom is. If your symptom happens too often to rate every time you do it, then your therapist and you will work out a specific time of day for you to keep track of it.

Symptom: _____

Date	Time	Obsession (or worry)	Compulsion	OCD thermometer (0–10)

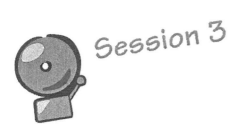 *Session 3*

Chapter

3

Review of Past Week

Starting in session 3 and continuing for all remaining sessions, you will spend a few minutes talking to your therapist about how you've been feeling since the last time you met with him or her. Fill in the blanks in the following form so you and your therapist can talk about what you did and any good things that might have happened to you.

What good things happened this week?

Write down one good thing that you did or that happened to you during the past week:

_____

_____

Write down one thing you did this week to fight your OCD:

_____

_____

Your First Exposure

Today you will participate in your first exposure exercise. You will work with your therapist to figure out which item from the My Symptom List will be the best one to start with. Sometimes, things that make kids feel anxious at home or school don't make them feel that way when they are in the office. So you may need to try a couple of different things to find the one that works the best for you. It will be like an experiment where you and your therapist are testing hypotheses or ideas.

There are a lot of different ways to do exposures. For example, if you are afraid of germs or touching dirty things, your therapist may ask you to touch something that isn't very clean and help you resist the urge to wash your hands right afterward. If one of your compulsions is to arrange your books or papers in a certain order, your therapist may ask you to mess them up on purpose and then resist the urge to fix them.

During the exposure, your therapist will pay careful attention to how you are feeling, and will ask you to use the OCD thermometer to rate how anxious or nervous you feel. It is important to pay careful attention to how the exposure exercise is done, because you will be asked to practice at home on your own. Your therapist will help you plan for your take-home practice and show you how to keep track of your OCD thermometer ratings using the Exposure Practice Form included here. One copy of this form is included for each week of the program. If you need extras, you may photocopy them from your workbook or download multiple copies from the companion Web site at www.oup.com/us/ttw.

Exercises

- On your own at home, practice the exposures you did during the session.

- Remember to graph your OCD thermometer ratings on the ERP Practice Form and bring it to the next session.

ERP Practice Form

Name: _____ Date: _____

Symptom: _____

_____

Exposure: _____

Ways to Fight OCD Thoughts: _____

_____

_____

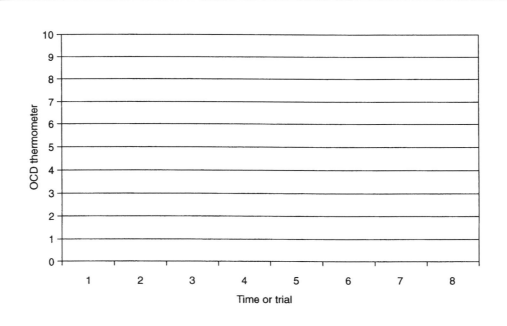

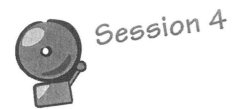 Session 4

Review of Past Week

As you did during your last session, you will spend a few minutes talking to your therapist about how you've been feeling since the last time you met with him or her. Once again, fill in the blanks in the following form so you and your therapist can talk about what you did and any good things that might have happened to you.

What good things happened this week?

Write down one good thing that you did or that happened to you during the past week:

_____

_____

Write down one thing you did this week to fight your OCD:

_____

_____

Next, you will fill out the Child/Adolescent Global Improvement Rating included here. This form will show you how much your OCD has improved since you started this program. It is a good way for you and your therapist to monitor your progress.

Child/Adolescent Global Improvement Rating

Name: _____ Date: _____

Circle the number that best describes how you feel your OCD has changed since the beginning of treatment.

1. Very much better   5. A little worse

2. Much better   6. Much worse

3. A little better   7. Very much worse

4. No change

Circle the number that best describes how you feel your overall functioning has changed since the beginning of treatment.

1. Very much better   5. A little worse

2. Much better   6. Much worse

3. A little better   7. Very much worse

4. No change

Comments: _____

_____

_____

Changing Your OCD Thoughts

Today, your therapist will teach you ways to help control the thoughts you have that make you want to do your rituals. You will talk about your OCD thoughts and come up with some more helpful thoughts you can use to fight your OCD. This is called *cognitive restructuring* and you can use it to feel less anxious during your exposure exercises.

For example, let's say that your OCD makes you think you are going to get sick if you don't wash your hands after touching a doorknob. A more helpful thought may be to think about how many other people have touched the same doorknob without getting sick. How many people do you know that have gotten sick from touching doorknobs? Probably, no one. Here are some questions you can ask yourself if your OCD makes you afraid to touch certain things:

"What are the chances that if I touch _____, I will get sick?"

"How many other people have touched _____ and have gotten sick?"

"Has everyone who has touched _____ become sick?"

Write down one of your OCD thoughts here:

_____

Can you think of some helpful thoughts you can use to fight this thought? List them here:

1. _____

2. _____

3. _____

Here are some other thoughts you can use to control your OCD:

- "This is just my OCD talking."

- "Nothing bad will happen if I don't do my ritual; it's just a false alarm."

- "I'm stronger than my OCD; I don't need to give in to it."

- "The more I resist giving in to my OCD, the weaker it will get."

Sometimes you are stronger than your OCD and other times your OCD seems stronger than you. Drawing pictures of your OCD can be another helpful way to fight it. First draw a picture of what your OCD looks like when it is stronger than you.

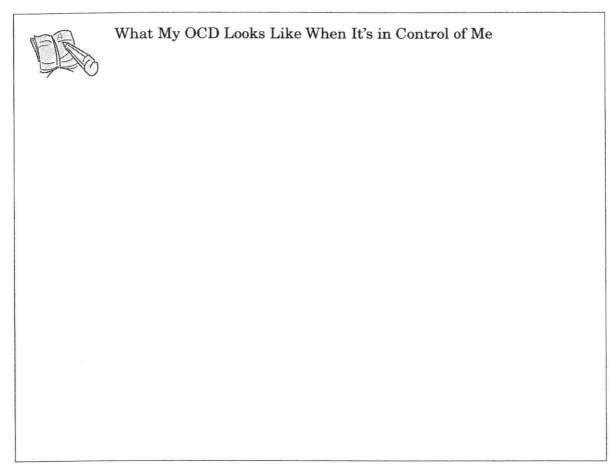

What My OCD Looks Like When It's in Control of Me

Next, draw a picture of what your OCD looks like when you are stronger.

What My OCD Looks Like When I'm in Control of It

When you are doing exposures, looking at or thinking about these pictures is another way to challenge your OCD thoughts. Sometimes thinking of a funny name for your OCD can also help. Think of a funny name to call your OCD and write it here:

Exposure Practice

During this session you will practice more exposure exercises. Remember the exercises from last session? This time you will probably practice with a symptom higher up on your symptom list.

During the exposure, your therapist will pay careful attention to how you are feeling and will ask you to use the OCD thermometer to rate how anxious or nervous you feel. Your therapist will remind you to use your helpful thoughts to fight your OCD thoughts so you will feel less anxious during the exposure.

Exercises

- On your own at home, practice the exposures you did during the session.

- Remember to graph your OCD thermometer ratings on the ERP Practice Form and bring it to the next session.

Name: _____ Date: _____

Symptom: _____

_____

Exposure: _____

Ways to Fight OCD Thoughts: _____

_____

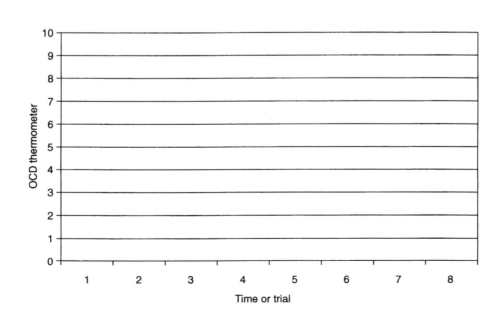

 Session 5

Chapter

5

Review of Past Week

As you did during your last session, you will spend a few minutes talking to your therapist about how you've been feeling since the last time you met with him or her. Once again, fill in the blanks in the following form so you and your therapist can talk about what you did and any good things that might have happened to you.

What good things happened this week?

Write down one good thing that you did or that happened to you during the past week:

_____

_____

Write down one thing you did this week to fight your OCD:

_____

_____

Rerate Your Symptom List

Today, you and your therapist will review the My Symptom List and rerate your symptoms using the OCD thermometer (see page 17). Some of the ratings you gave to your symptoms at the beginning of this program may be different now.

Use the My Symptom List to add any new symptoms you may have noticed since starting treatment and write your new ratings in the column for session 5.

It may be that some of the symptoms you have been working on in session and at home may be less upsetting or easier to resist compared with the beginning of the program. If so, this is a sign that your hard work is paying off. You are getting stronger and your OCD is getting weaker! However, for some people, it can take a little bit more time to see these changes. If your symptom ratings didn't change, you and your therapist can talk about what else you might do to work on these items.

Exposure Practice

After you have updated your symptom list, you and your therapist will choose the next exposure item to start working on. During the exposure, your therapist will pay careful attention to how you are feeling and will ask you to use the OCD thermometer to rate how anxious or nervous you feel. Your therapist will remind you to use your helpful thoughts to fight your OCD thoughts so you will feel less anxious during the exposure.

OCD Thoughts

Did you know that everybody has bothersome and unwanted thoughts? In fact, people without OCD have the same types and number of thoughts as people with OCD. The big difference is that people without OCD don't pay attention to all of these thoughts the way that people with OCD do. Instead of getting upset by unwanted thoughts or images, most people just treat them like background noise—like if the TV is on somewhere but you are not watching it. You may hear the sound, but most of the time you don't even know what is being said. Unfortunately, people with OCD are often more sensitive to their thoughts and have a harder time ignoring them.

Remember we talked about fighting your OCD thoughts during session 4? As we said then, we call this *cognitive restructuring,* and it can also be used to help you with you unwanted thoughts or images. Let's say that some of your OCD thoughts or images make you feel bad about yourself—maybe because you know these thoughts don't make any sense, but you are still scared by them. Or maybe you feel bad because you don't think these thoughts are appropriate or "right" and you don't think you should be having them. One way you can try to make yourself feel better is by thinking of some helpful thoughts instead. For example, you can remind yourself that the OCD thoughts aren't really true and don't mean anything about you or anyone else. They are just random noises playing in the background—like the TV, radio, or your MP3 player. Or you can remind yourself that everyone—not just people with OCD—has scary, embarrassing, or silly thoughts and images at different times, and these thoughts are nothing special. Remember, this is just your OCD talking to you and trying to trick you into thinking something bad is going to happen. But instead of being real, you know these thoughts are only a false alarm! You can talk back to your OCD and tell it you are not going to fall for that old trick again!

My Symptom List

Name: _____

OCD Thermometer Rating

DATE:					
SESSION:	1	5			
SYMPTOM:					

Pick one OCD thought or image to practice talking back to and write it down here:

_____

Now write down some things you could you say to your OCD thought or image so it doesn't make you feel so bad or so you don't have to pay so much attention to it:

1. _____

2. _____

3. _____

Facing Your OCD Thoughts and Images

There are a lot of different ways to help make your OCD thoughts stop bothering you so much. You can think them in your head, tell them to your therapist, write them down or draw pictures of them, read the descriptions or show the pictures to your therapist or other people, have your therapist read the description back to you, or sing or rap the thought. You may not realize it, but these are all different kinds of exposures—just like the exposures you and your therapist have already been doing, only you will do these with thoughts instead of behaviors. You and your therapist may even be able to think up some other exposures you can do to make your OCD thoughts bother you less.

For most kids, it's best to start with the easiest thing you can do first and then work your way up to more difficult exposures. The first thing is to decide the best place to start.

Write the OCD thought you are going to work on here:

_____

The following list contains a number of different ways you can expose this thought. There are a few blank spaces at the bottom in case you and your therapist come up with some additional ideas. Now rank the exposures in order from easiest to hardest, starting with the number 1.

Rank (1 is easiest)	Exposure List
_____	Imagine the thought
_____	Write the thought
_____	Draw a picture of the thought
_____	Say the thought out loud
_____	Tell the thought to my therapist
_____	Show my therapist a picture of the thought
_____	Have my therapist read my description of the thought
_____	Sing the thought
_____	Record the thought and listen to it
_____	_____
_____	_____

After you've ranked the different ways to expose your OCD thoughts, you can start with the easiest exposure first. Keep track of your OCD thermometer ratings on your ERP Practice Form. The goal is to practice each exposure until you can do it without feeling anxious. Remember to use your helping thoughts to talk back to your OCD.

Exercises

■ On your own at home, practice the exposures you did during the session.

■ Remember to graph your OCD thermometer ratings on the ERP Practice Form and bring it to the next session.

Name: _____ Date: _____

Symptom: _____

_____

Exposure: _____

Ways to Fight OCD Thoughts: _____

_____

_____

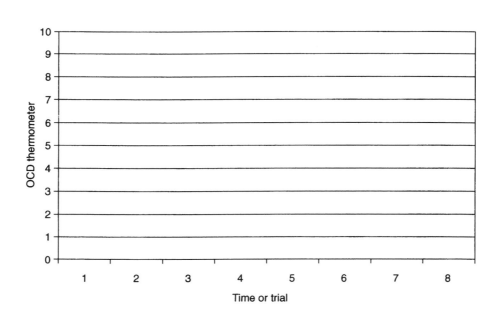

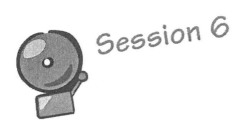 Session 6

Chapter
6

Review of Past Week

As you did during your last session, you will spend a few minutes talking to your therapist about how you've been feeling since the last time you met with him or her. Once again, fill in the following form so you and your therapist can talk about what you did and any good things that might have happened to you.

What good things happened this week?

Write down one good thing that you did or that happened to you during the past week:

_____

_____

Write down one thing you did this week to fight your OCD:

_____

_____

Exposure Practice

Today you and your therapist will start by reviewing the exercises you did at home during the past week. Then you will practice more exposures.

Beginning to Look Ahead

How are you feeling at this point in the program? This is a good time to review all the exposures you have been doing and to look back over what you have accomplished. You will continue to move up the symptom list each week, so remember to use all of your progress so far to help you face the upcoming exposures, too.

Are you still having some trouble with some of the items you've been working on? If so, your therapist will work with you to do some "touch-up exercises" to help make these exposures go more smoothly. Go ahead and practice these exercises with your therapist in session. As in every session, during the exposures your therapist will pay careful attention to how you are feeling and will ask you to use the OCD thermometer to rate how anxious or nervous you feel. Your therapist will remind you to use your helpful thoughts to fight your OCD thoughts so you will feel less anxious during the exposure.

Picture of Your OCD

During session 4 you drew a picture of what your OCD looks like when it has control over you. Now is a good time to draw a picture of what your OCD looks like at this point in your treatment. But this time, also include yourself in the picture and show how you are going to beat your OCD. You can draw this any way you want—perhaps you can be a superhero and your OCD is a villain, or you can draw yourself outsmarting your OCD in some way. The most important thing is to use your imagination.

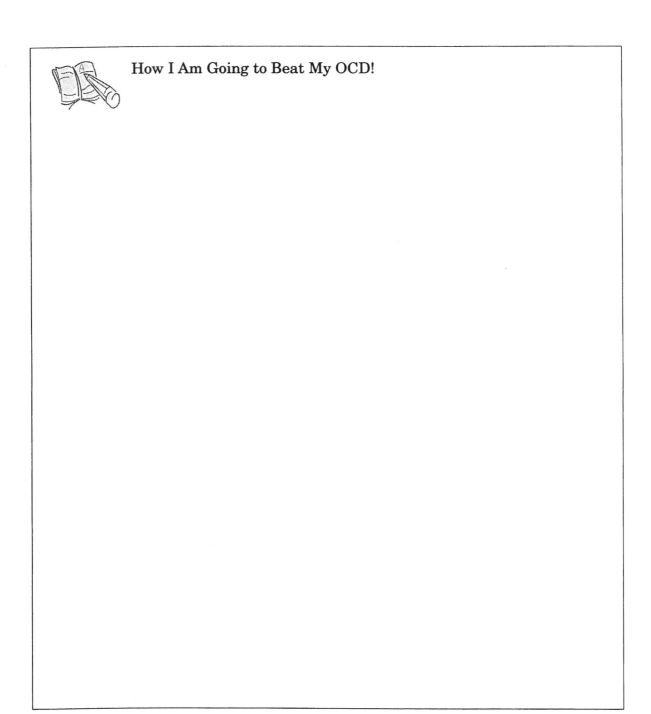

How I Am Going to Beat My OCD!

Exercises

■ On your own at home, practice the exposures you did during the session.

■ Remember to graph your OCD thermometer ratings on the ERP Practice Form and bring it to the next session.

Name: _____ Date: _____

Symptom: _____

_____

Exposure: _____

Ways to Fight OCD Thoughts: _____

_____

_____

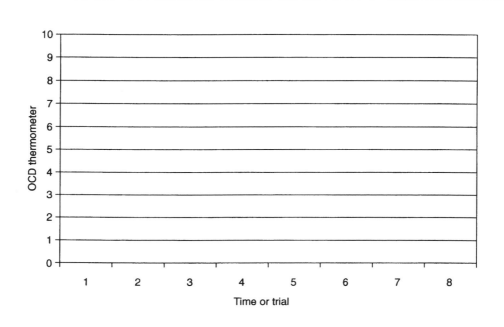

 Session 7

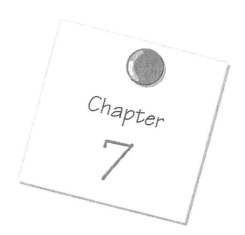
Chapter
7

Review of Past Week

As you did during your last session, you will spend a few minutes talking to your therapist about how you've been feeling since the last time you met with him or her. Once again, fill in the following form so you and your therapist can talk about what you did and any good things that might have happened to you.

What good things happened this week?

Write down one good thing that you did or that happened to you during the past week:

_____

_____

Write down one thing you did this week to fight your OCD:

_____

_____

Rerate Your Symptom List

Today, you and your therapist will review the My Symptom List you revised in session 5. Your therapist will ask you to rerate your symptoms using the OCD thermometer (see page 17). Use the My Symptom List to add any new symptoms you may have noticed since starting treatment and write your new ratings in the column for session 7.

Like last time, you might notice that some of your symptom ratings are lower now. If so, this is a sign that your hard work is paying off. You are getting stronger and your OCD is getting weaker! However, for some people, it can take a little bit more time to see these changes. If your symptom ratings didn't change as much as you would like, you and your therapist can talk about what else you might do to work on these items. Keep up your hard work and focus on the progress you have made so far!

Exposure Practice

After you update your symptom list, you will review with your therapist the exercises you have been doing at home in between sessions. Then you will practice more exposures. Keep moving up your symptom list and practice the items that have higher ratings. During the exposures, your therapist will pay careful attention to how you are feeling and will ask you to use the OCD thermometer to rate how anxious or nervous you feel. Your therapist will remind you to use your helpful thoughts to fight your OCD thoughts so you will feel less anxious during the exposure.

Preparing for Harder Exposures

Like we talked about during the last session, you are starting to practice harder and harder exposures. Be confident and look at how far you've come! You will be able to handle facing your OCD items one step at a time. Your therapist will help you.

▦ On your own at home, practice the exposures you did during the session.

▦ Remember to graph your OCD thermometer ratings on the ERP Practice Form and bring it to the next session.

My Symptom List

Name: _____

OCD Thermometer Rating

DATE:					
SESSION:	1	5	7		
SYMPTOM:					

ERP Practice Form

Name: _____ Date: _____

Symptom: _____

_____

Exposure: _____

Ways to Fight OCD Thoughts: _____

_____

_____

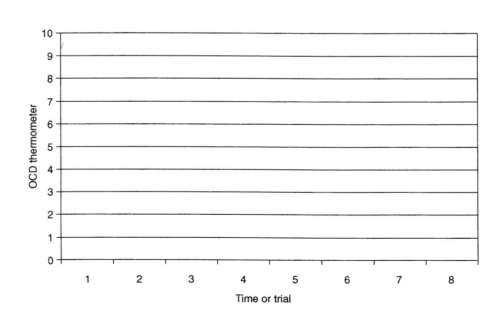

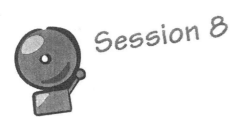 

Session 8

Review of Past Week

As you did during your last session, you will spend a few minutes talking to your therapist about how you've been feeling since the last time you met with him or her. Once again, fill in the following form so you and your therapist can talk about what you did and any good things that may have happened to you.

> **What good things happened this week?**
>
> Write down one good thing that you did or that happened to you during the past week:
>
> _____
>
> _____
>
> Write down one thing you did this week to fight your OCD:
>
> _____
>
> _____

Next, you will fill out the Child/Adolescent Global Improvement Rating once again. Remember, this form will show you how much better your OCD has gotten since you started this program.

Child/Adolescent Global Improvement Rating

Name: _____ Date: _____

Circle the number that best describes how you feel your OCD has changed since the beginning of treatment.

1. Very much better   5. A little worse

2. Much better   6. Much worse

3. A little better   7. Very much worse

4. No change

Circle the number that best describes how you feel your overall functioning has changed since the beginning of treatment.

1. Very much better   5. A little worse

2. Much better   6. Much worse

3. A little better   7. Very much worse

4. No change

Comments: _____

_____

_____

Exposure Practice

Today you will review with your therapist the exercises you completed at home. Then you will practice exposing yourself to symptoms that you rated higher on the OCD thermometer.

During the exposures, your therapist will pay careful attention to how you are feeling and will ask you to use the OCD thermometer to rate how anxious or nervous you feel. Your therapist will remind you to use your helpful thoughts to fight your OCD thoughts so you will feel less anxious during the exposure.

Starting Harder Exposures

At this point in the program, you may already be working on symptoms higher up on the symptom list you created. This is when you really have to gear yourself up to do battle with your OCD. Because you have been practicing the lower items on your list, the higher items may not seem quite as hard any more. Your therapist will help you break down each of these new exposures into easier, smaller steps if necessary. Also, the tools you have learned so far will continue to help you as you work your way up the list.

 Write down some of the things that have helped you fight your OCD so far:

1. _____

2. _____

(continued on next page)

3. _____

4. _____

5. _____

Exercises

▨ On your own at home, practice the exposures you did during the session.

▨ Remember to graph your OCD thermometer ratings on the ERP Practice Form and bring it to the next session.

ERP Practice Form

Name: _____ Date: _____

Symptom: _____

_____

Exposure: _____

Ways to Fight OCD Thoughts: _____

_____

_____

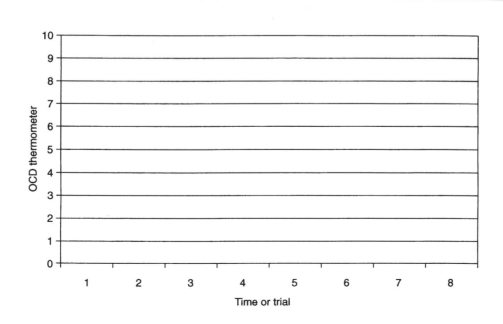

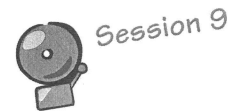 Session 9

 Chapter 9

Review of Past Week

As you did during your last session, you will spend a few minutes talking to your therapist about how you've been feeling since the last time you met with him or her. Once again, fill in the following form so you and your therapist can talk about what you did and any good things that might have happened to you.

What good things happened this week?

Write down one good thing that you did or that happened to you during the past week:

_____

_____

Write down one thing you did this week to fight your OCD:

_____

_____

_____

Rerate Your Symptom List

Today, you and your therapist will review the My Symptom List you revised during session 7. Your therapist will ask you to rerate your symptoms using the OCD thermometer (see page 17). Use the My Symptom List to add any new symptoms you may have noticed since starting treatment and write your new ratings in the column for session 9.

By now, some of your ratings are probably getting lower. How does that make you feel? Do you see the progress you are making? You are doing great and getting stronger while your OCD is getting weaker!

Are you still having some trouble with some of the items you've been working on? For some people, it can take longer to see these changes. If your symptom ratings didn't change as much as you'd like, you and your therapist can talk about what else you might do to work on these items.

Exposure Practice

After you update your symptom list, you will review with your therapist the exercises you have been doing at home in between sessions. Then you will practice exposures with the next item on your list. Remember to use the cognitive restructuring techniques you have learned if these more difficult exposures make you feel extra scared or anxious.

During the exposures, your therapist will pay careful attention to how you are feeling and will ask you to use the OCD thermometer to rate how anxious or nervous you feel. Your therapist will remind you to use your helpful thoughts to fight your OCD thoughts so you will feel less anxious during the exposure.

Planning for the End of the Program

Now that you have been working on your OCD for several weeks, your therapist may want to talk to you about the end of the program.

My Symptom List

Name: _____

OCD Thermometer Rating

DATE:					
SESSION:	1	5	7	9	
SYMPTOM:					

What do you think about the progress you have made? How do you feel about completing this program? Do you have any worries or fears about what will happen after treatment? Use the space provided to write about your feelings about ending the program.

_____

_____

_____

_____

Use the space provided to write down any questions that you want to ask your therapist or anything you want to discuss with your therapist before the program ends.

1. _____

2. _____

3. _____

4. _____

5. _____

- On your own at home, practice the exposures you did during the session.

- Remember to graph your OCD thermometer ratings on the ERP Practice Form and bring it to the next session.

Name: _____ Date: _____

Symptom: _____

_____

Exposure: _____

Ways to Fight OCD Thoughts: _____

_____

_____

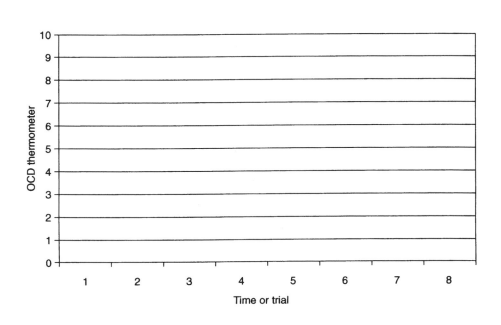

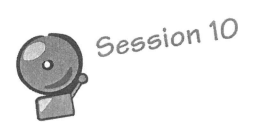 Session 10

Chapter

10

Review of Past Week

As you did during your last session, you will spend a few minutes talking to your therapist about how you've been feeling since the last time you met with him or her. Once again, fill in the following form so you and your therapist can talk about what you did and any good things that might have happened to you.

What good things happened this week?

Write down one good thing that you did or that happened to you during the past week:

_____

_____

Write down one thing you did this week to fight your OCD:

_____

_____

Exposure Practice

Today you will review with your therapist the exercises you did at home. Then you will practice more exposures with some of the highest remaining symptoms on the My Symptom List you created.

Once again, during the exposures your therapist will pay careful attention to how you are feeling and will ask you to use the OCD thermometer to rate how anxious or nervous you feel. Your therapist will remind you to use your helpful thoughts to fight your OCD thoughts so you will feel less anxious during the exposure.

Fighting OCD After the Program Ends

At this point in the program, you may only have a few sessions left. By now you have learned a number of tools to help you control and cope with your OCD. You can continue to use these tools after the program has ended. One way to practice using these tools is to pretend that you are a therapist who is helping someone else with OCD. If someone came to you for help with their OCD, what would you do to help them? Let's start at the beginning.

First, how would you explain OCD to this person?

Write down two OCD symptoms for this person. Try to use symptoms that you have had but not yet worked on in treatment or that you haven't had yourself but you think may come up in the future:

Symptom 1: _____

Symptom 2: _____

The next step is to come up with exposures and helpful thoughts for each of these symptoms. You can do this using the ERP Practice Forms provided on the next two pages. Complete an ERP Practice Form for each symptom. After you've come up with exposures and helping thoughts for each symptom, fill in the graph on each practice form to show how well you think these exposures will work for this person.

Great job! You can use this same strategy to deal with any OCD symptoms that might start to bother you after you have completed the program.

Living Life Without OCD

One of the worst things about having OCD is the way it can mess things up at school, with friends, with family, or at home. For most kids, however, having their OCD get better also means that things at home, at school, and with other people also improve. Is this true for you as well? Take a minute to think about the things that your OCD used to make it hard for you to do. Now think about how that has changed.

ERP Practice Form

Name: _____ Date: _____

Symptom: _____

_____

Exposure: _____

Ways to Fight OCD Thoughts: _____

_____

_____

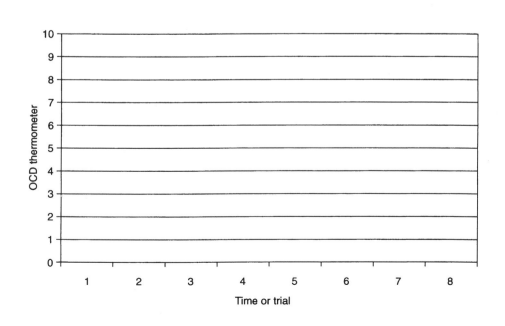

Name: _____ Date: _____

Symptom: _____

_____

Exposure: _____

Ways to Fight OCD Thoughts: _____

_____

_____

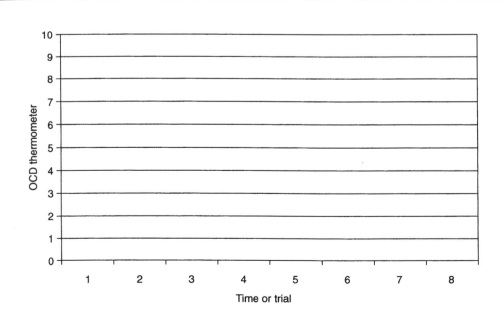

Write down some things that you can now do that used to be hard because of your OCD:

1._____

2._____

3._____

4._____

5._____

If you were able to list some things on this list, that is a good sign that you are getting stronger and your OCD is getting weaker. Congratulations! Your hard work is really paying off! For some kids, however, it can take longer for things at home, at school, or with other people to get better. If so, it's important that you keep working in treatment. Your therapist will work with you to come up with some ways to help things get better in these areas. Although it may take a little longer, the more you keep fighting your OCD, the better things will get for you.

Exercises

■ On your own at home, practice the exposures you did during the session.

■ Remember to graph your OCD thermometer ratings on the ERP Practice Form and bring it to the next session.

Name: _____ Date: _____

Symptom: _____

_____

Exposure: _____

Ways to Fight OCD Thoughts: _____

_____

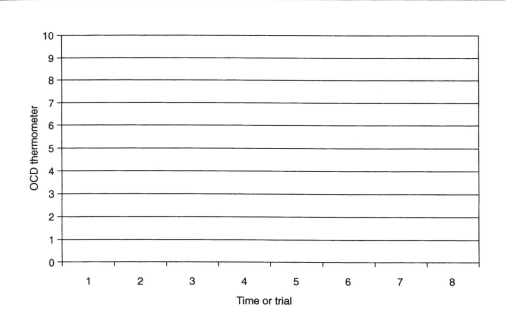

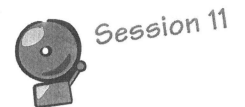 *Session 11*

Chapter

11

Review of Past Week

As you did during your last session, you will spend a few minutes talking to your therapist about how you've been feeling since the last time you met with him or her. Once again, fill in the following form so you and your therapist can talk about what you did and any good things that might have happened to you.

What good things happened this week?

Write down one good thing that you did or that happened to you during the past week:

_____

_____

Write down one thing you did this week to fight your OCD:

_____

_____

Rerate Your Symptom List

At the beginning of this session, you and your therapist will review the My Symptom List and rerate your symptoms using the OCD thermometer (see page 17). Use the My Symptom List to add any new symptoms you may have noticed since starting treatment and write your new ratings in the column for session 11.

By now, most of your symptoms may have much lower ratings than they did at the beginning of the program. This wouldn't be possible if it wasn't for all of your effort. You worked really hard and should be very proud of yourself.

How does that make you feel? Do you see the progress you are making? You are doing great and getting stronger while your OCD is getting weaker!

Are you still having some trouble with some of the symptoms you've been working on? For some people, it can take longer to see these changes. If your symptom ratings didn't change as much as you'd like, you and your therapist can talk about what else you might do to work on these items.

Exposure Practice

You will start session 11 like you have started all the other sessions. You will review with your therapist the practice exercises you did at home on your own. Then you will practice the last of your most difficult exposures.

Once again, your therapist will pay careful attention to how you are reacting during the exposure and will ask you to let him or her know how you are feeling. Remember to use the numbers from the OCD thermometer to tell your therapist how anxious or nervous you feel. Also, remember to use your helpful thoughts to fight your OCD and help you feel less anxious during your exposure practice.

My Symptom List

Name: _____

OCD Thermometer Rating

DATE:					
SESSION:	1	5	7	9	11
SYMPTOM:					

Planning for Graduation

Your therapist will talk to you about your upcoming graduation from the program. Is there anything special you would like to do to celebrate? Write down your ideas for your graduation on the lines provided.

My Graduation:

_____

_____

_____

_____

_____

Fighting OCD After the Program Ends

You and your therapist will continue talking about ways to deal with any OCD symptoms that might start to bother you again after treatment ends. Remember your last session, when you were the therapist and you created practice forms to help someone else with OCD? Do you have any questions about how to do this for yourself if the need arises? If so, you and your therapist can practice creating some new exposure plans today. If there is anything else you want to ask your therapist about OCD, or any of the exposures you have done in treatment, or about how to cope with your OCD once the program ends, now is a good time to ask.

If you have any questions, you can write them down here:

_____

_____

_____

_____

Exercises

■ On your own at home, practice the exposures you did during the session.

■ Remember to graph your OCD thermometer ratings on the ERP Practice Form and bring it to the next session.

Name: _____   Date: _____

Symptom: _____

_____

Exposure: _____

Ways to Fight OCD Thoughts: _____

_____

_____

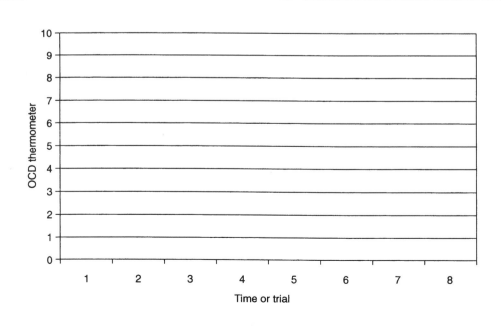

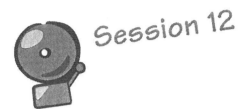 Session 12

 Chapter 12

Review of Past Week

As you have done all along, you will spend a few minutes talking to your therapist about how you've been feeling since the last time you met with him or her. For the last time, fill in the following form so you and your therapist can talk about what you did and any good things that might have happened to you.

What good things happened this week?

Write down one good thing that you did or that happened to you during the past week:

_____

_____

Write down one thing you did this week to fight your OCD:

_____

_____

Exposure Practice

Today you will review with your therapist the exercises you did at home. Then you will practice exposures for any symptoms still remaining on your symptom list. If you have already done exposures with all the symptoms on your list, your therapist may want to review with you some of the past exposures you have done during treatment. This is a good way to see the progress you have made in the program. Reviewing the things you worked on in treatment is also a good way to help you remember the tools you learned in case you need to use them again in the future.

Fighting OCD After the Program Ends

Today you will again practice being the therapist and helping someone else who has OCD. However, this time the person you help will be your therapist! You and your therapist will switch places. You will pretend to be your therapist and your therapist will pretend to be someone with OCD. Are you ready? Your therapist will tell you about two OCD symptoms that have been bothering him or her. Write the two OCD symptoms here:

Symptom 1: _____

Symptom 2: _____

Now complete an ERP Practice Form for each of these symptoms. Pick one of the symptoms and have your therapist practice doing the exposure you created.

ERP Practice Form

Name: _____ Date: _____

Symptom: _____

_____

Exposure: _____

Ways to Fight OCD Thoughts: _____

_____

_____

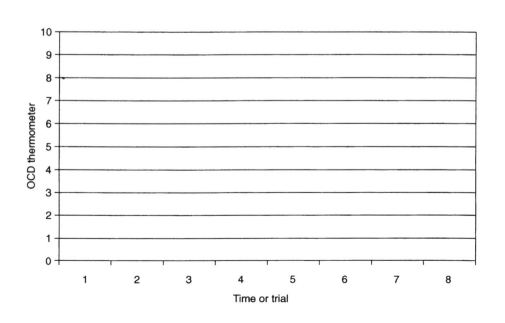

Name: _____ Date: _____

Symptom: _____

_____

Exposure: _____

Ways to Fight OCD Thoughts: _____

_____

_____

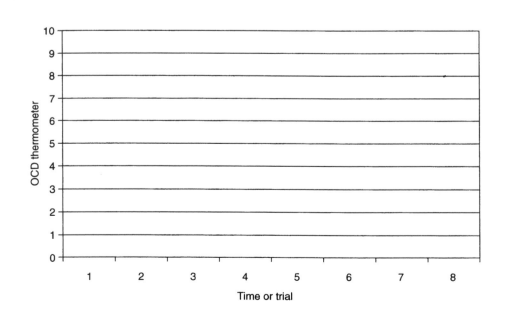

Congratulations! You have successfully completed the program and are now ready to manage your OCD on your own.

Congratulations!

_____

has successfully completed the "It's Only a False Alarm" program!

Date: _____

Therapist: _____

Congratulations!

_____

has successfully completed the "It's Only a False Alarm" program!

Date: _____

Therapist: _____